LIFE
The most important game you'll ever play

Beverly D. Schaefgen

LIfe
The most important game you'll ever play

by Beverly D. Schaefgen

ISBN-13: 978-1725941526
ISBN-10: 172594152X

©2018 Beverly D. Schaefgen

The quotes by famous people were borrowed according to fair use law and attributed.

Cover artwork by J. Michael Schaefgen
Original artwork by J. Michael Schaefgen

Published by Monument Press 2018
Printed by CreateSpace

A division of
Bluff City Communications Inc.
books@bluffcitycomm.com

Contents

Self-Care..1

Self-Talk 7

Self-Definition 15

Self-Success 23

Self-Sacrifice..35

Self-Destruction 43

Self-Forgiveness 49

Self-Control...57

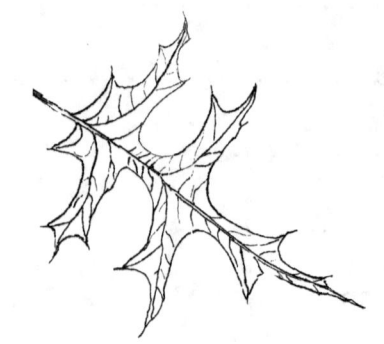

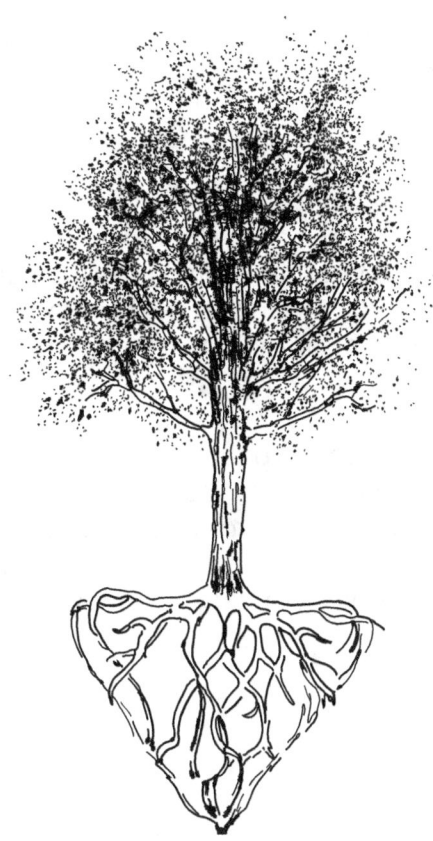

Self-Care

The art of treating yourself with loving care.

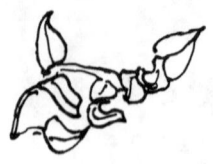

It has been my experience that GOD *always* wins! This simply means the sooner one walks the path GOD intents for them, the sooner they will experience a more meaningful life and begin to feel more fulfilled in their life.

Realize you teach the people in your lives how to treat you by either accepting or not accepting their negative behavior towards you as well as by modeling how you treat yourself. Think of it this way, why should someone else treat you better than you treat yourself?

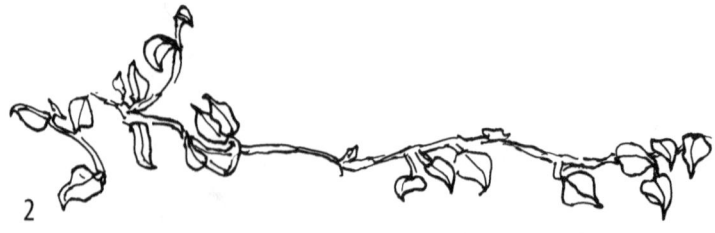

"Someday, when I manage to finally figure out how to take care of myself, then I'll consider taking care of someone else."

~Marilyn Monroe

"You cannot hope to build a better world without improving the individuals. To that end, each of us must work for his own improvement and, at the same time, share a general responsibility for all humanity, our particular duty being to aid those to whom we think we can be most useful."

~Marie Curie

"There are three kinds of men. The ones that learn by reading. The few who learn by observation. The rest of them have to pee on the electric fence for themselves."

~Will Rogers

"In order to change the world, you have to get your head together first."

– Jimi Hendrix

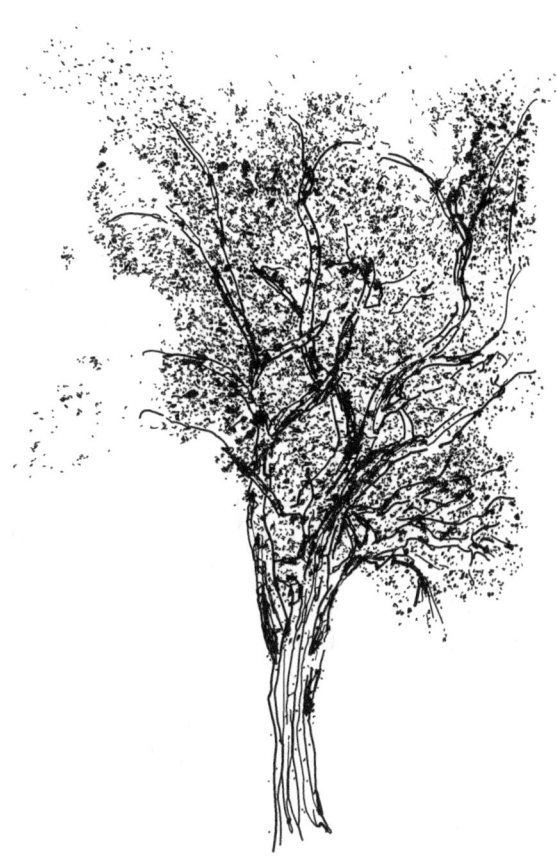

Self-Talk

The habit of speaking to and about yourself with loving respect.

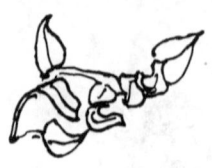

You're always communicating with the Universe through your thoughts, your words, your actions and your deeds. The information you send out into the Universe is returned to you in kind. In other words, whether you're communicating positively or negatively, the Universe can only response to you in the same vibration. It is for this reason that monitoring your thoughts and your words is of upmost importance to your well-being. Your thoughts and your words have the ability to alter your actions and your deeds, which will positively or negatively impact the quality of your life.

Perception is everything. If you perceive (believe) something as a positive in your life, then it is a positive. Conversely, if you perceive (believe) something to be negative in your life, then it is negative.

We all have that relative and/or friend who constantly focuses on what they consider their faults or shortcomings. Nothing in their life is right enough, good enough, fair or just enough. Such negative talk sent out into the Universe can only be answered in the same vibration. So, this relative and/or friend will continue to experience negativity because of their thoughts, their words, their actions and their deeds. Get it?

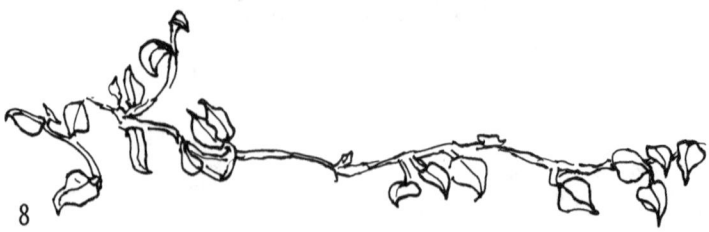

"Things are products of your thinking. By thinking you are creating your life experiences. Think your desires into Creation."

Beverly D. Schaefgen

"Remember happiness doesn't depend upon who you are or what you have; it depends solely on what you think."

Dale Carnegie

> **"None but ourselves can free our minds."**
>
> *Bob Marley*

"Open your eyes, look within. Are you satisfied with the life your living?"

Bob Marley

"Every great work, every big accomplishment, has been brought into manifestation through holding to the vision, and often just before the big achievement, comes apparent failure and discouragement."

Florence Scovel Shinn

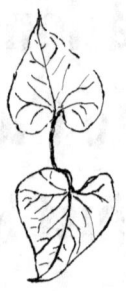

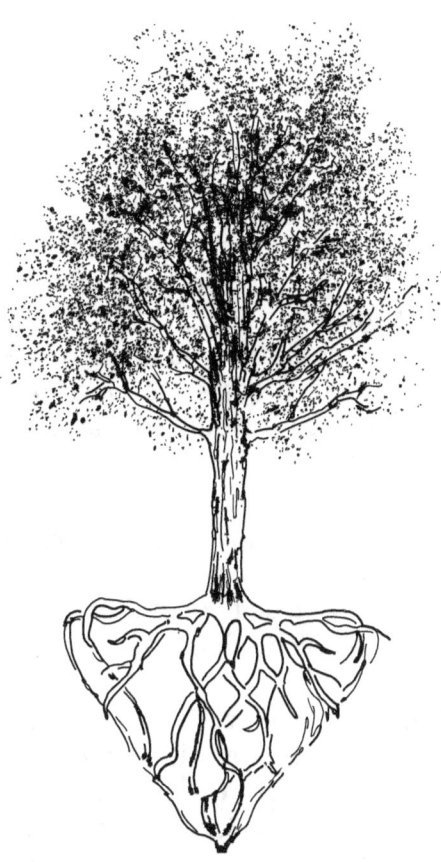

Self-Definition

The determination to always define yourself.

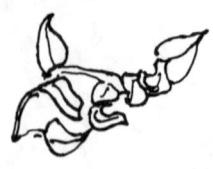

The government, society as a whole, family members, friends, employers and co-workers are prepared to assign you a definition or a label if you're unwilling, or intimated, or afraid to define yourself. Ask yourself if you are prepared to live a life that has been assigned to you. Or would you rather live a life you defined for yourself?

Every word you say, every decision you make or do not make, every action you take or do not take is a choice. Even if you decide to do nothing, you have still made a choice. A choice of inaction is still a choice.

Become the Chief Emotional Officer (CEO) of your own life. Everyone is responsible for their own emotional well-being. Take the time to recognize and understand your emotional response to every experience in your life. Ask yourself how interaction with a particular person or a particular group of people makes you feel. Do you feel happy, sad, mad, glad?

Remember that no one can make you feel anything that you don't first allow. Yes, your life is truly all about you.

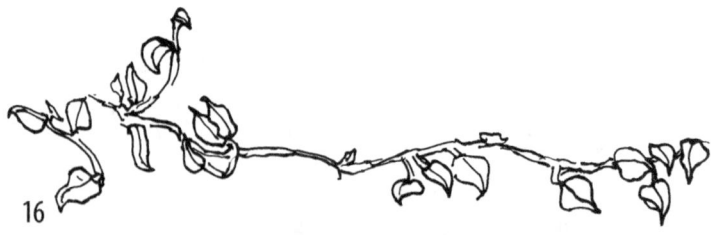

Be in charge of your day. Every day presents you with challenges. Consider thinking of these as learning experiences rather than as day-busters. By re-framing your daily experiences in this manner, you empower yourself.

People who feel empowered are confident in their abilities and they expect to succeed even if they stumble a few times alone the journey to achieving their ultimate goals. These people are the masters of their lives, they are the CEOs of their emotional state.

> "I am not what happened to me, I am what I choose to become."
>
> *Carl Jung*

"You need to overcome the tug of people against you as you reach for high goals."

George S. Patton

> "It is not necessary for eagles to be crows."
>
> — Sitting Bull

"Don't ever empty the bucket of mystery. Never let people define what you do. It's not about doing something unprecedented and unpredictable. It's just about never being a word, or something that is not the process of transformation."

Marilyn Monroe

"I've been imitated so well I've heard people copy my mistakes."

Jimi Hendrix

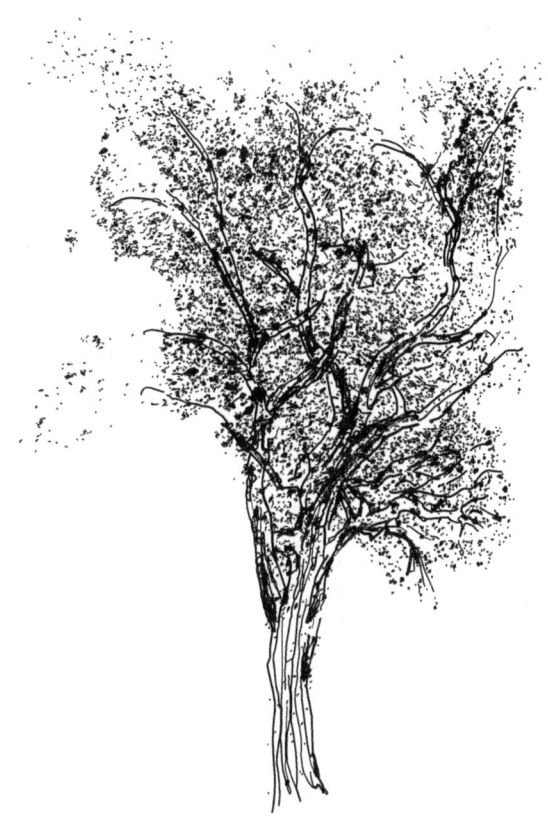

Self-Success

The journey that leads to your desired goal usually involves at least several missteps, tumbles and a couple of stumbles. Like a baby taking thier first steps, ultimately they find thier land legs and are off and running.

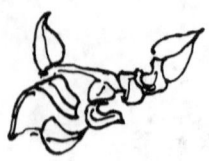

The concept of an overnight success is a myth. Rather success is a process involving a sort of dance, a few steps forward followed by several steps backwards, then repeat, until the forward momentum is strong enough to overpower the pull of the backward motion. Then instant success is achieved!

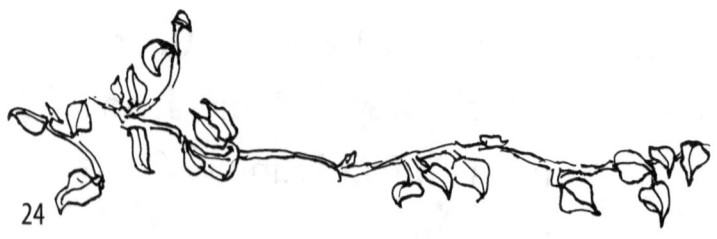

"The difference between where you are now and where you want to be is only the width between your ears."

Beverly D. Schaefgen

> "Success is a journey, not a destination. The doing is often more important than the outcome."
>
> *Arthur Ashe*

"Success is how high you bounce when you hit bottom."

George S. Patton

"Develop success from failures. Discouragement and failure are two of the surest stepping stones to success."

Dale Carnegie

"If you could kick the person in the pants responsible for most of your trouble, you wouldn't sit for a month."

Theodore Roosevelt

> "In the time of darkest defeat, victory may be nearest."
>
> — *William McKinley*

"We must dare to be great; and we must realize that greatness is the fruit of toil and sacrifice and high courage."

William H. Taft

"It is amazing what you can accomplish if you do not care who gets the credit."

Harry S. Truman

"Remember, always give your best. Never get discouraged. Never be petty. Always remember, others may hate you. But those who hate you don't win unless you hate them. And then you destroy yourself."

Richard M. Nixon

"Never be satisfied with less than your best effort. If you strive for the top and miss, you'll still beat the pack."

Gerald R. Ford

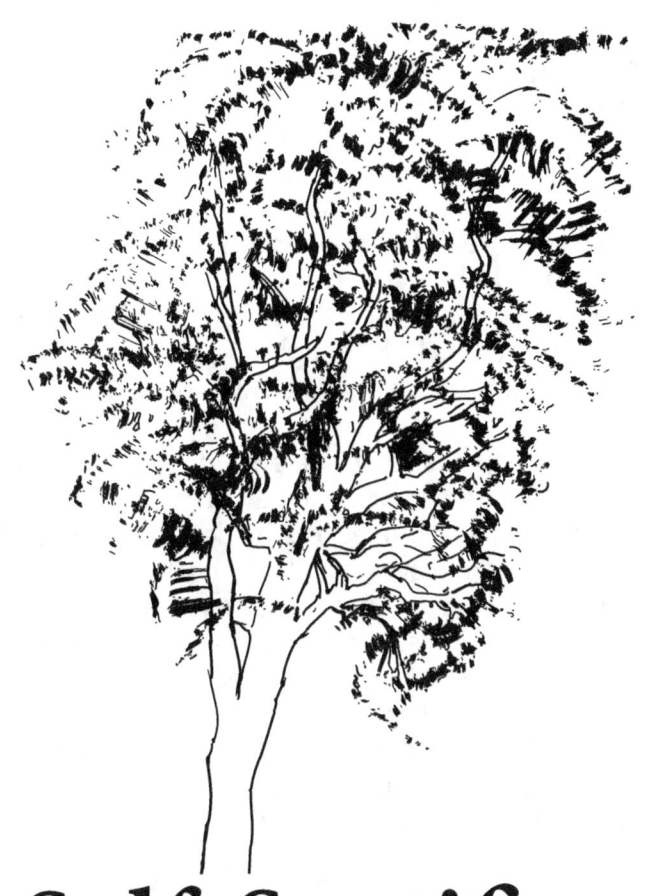

Self-Sacrifice

Deferring your own interests for the benefit of others or a for a cause.

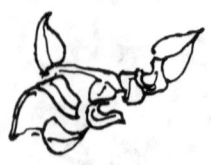

Some individuals have been taught or have developed a habit of abandoning their own interests or well-being for the benefit of others or for a cause. This typically is thought of as a noble deed; in reality, it drains the spirit from the giver.

It is of vital importance for parents to temporarily put their dreams aside in order to devote their time and the family's resources to provide for and raise their children. However, it is also important for parents to continue with their own education and spiritual growth. That being said, there is absolutely nothing negative about being helpful or considerate to others as along as you feel you are first being true to yourself. It's important to understand that successful persons are better able to mentor others because of their achievements and life experience.

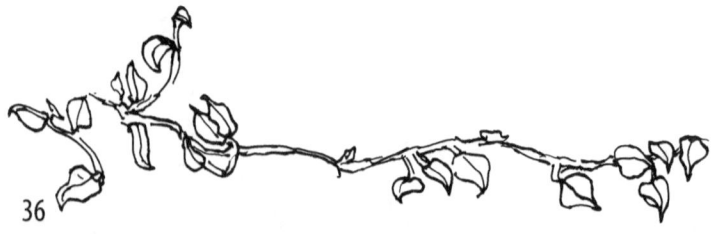

"Self-sacrifice enables us to sacrifice other people without blushing."
George Bernard Shaw

"Behold I do not give lectures or a little charity when I give of myself."

Walt Whitman

"The men and women who have the right ideals… are those who have the courage to strive for the happiness which comes only with labor and effort and self-sacrifice, and those whose joy in life springs in part from power of work and sense of duty."

Theodore Roosevelt

"Human progress is neither automatic nor inevitable… Every step toward the goal of justice requires sacrifice, suffering, and struggle; the tireless exertions and passionate concern of dedicated individuals."

Martin Luther King, Jr.

"Football is a great deal like life in that it teaches that work, sacrifice, perseverance, competitive drive, selflessness and respect for authority is the price that each and every one of us must pay to achieve any goal that is worthwhile."

Vince Lombardi

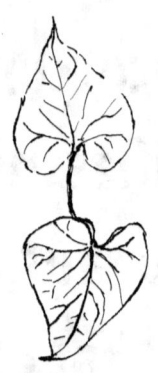

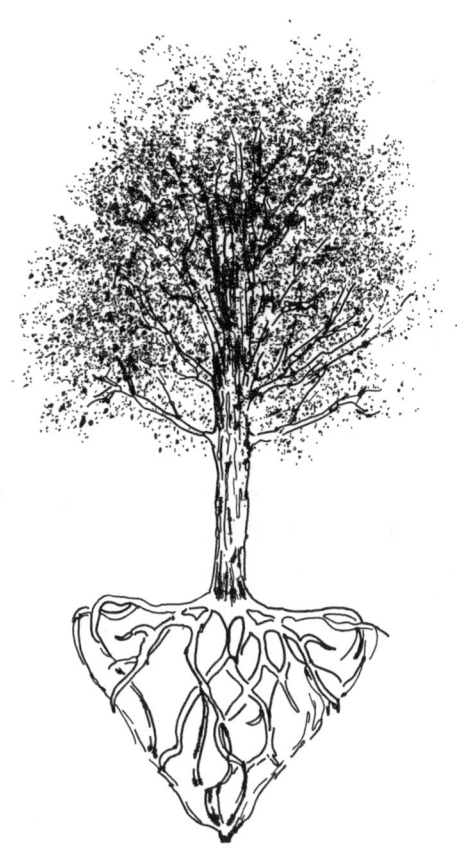

Self-Destruction

Self-harm can be thought of as a cry for help that if ignored by others may ultimately consume the individual.

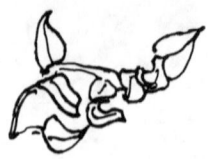

Self-destruction can take many forms such as substance abuse, eating disorders, gambling addictions, shopping addictions, sex addictions, etc. The ultimate form is suicide, which is frequently unexpected and totally irreversible.

The government invests billions of dollars a year to treat those suffering with various addictions. Addiction is a cruel disease that steals whatever it can from the addict leaving a wide swath of destruction in its path, ripping lives and families apart.

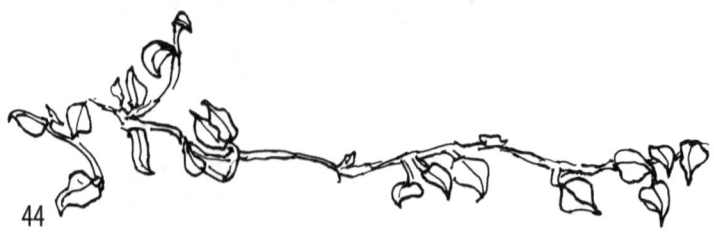

"In the past, destruction of your neighbor might have been considered a victory, but today we are all interdependent. We live in a global economy; we face problems like climate change that affect us all. The seven billion human beings alive today belong to one human family. In the context that others' interest are in our interest and our interest is in their interest, the use of force is self-destructive."

Dalai Lama

> "Self-destruction is the effect of cowardice in the highest extreme."
>
> — *Daniel Defoe*

"The human body is not a thing or substance, given, but a continuous creation. The human body is an energy system which is never a complete structure; never static; is in perpetual inner self-construction and self-destruction; we destroy in order to make it new."

Norman O. Brown

"In rock stardom there's an absolute economic upside to self-destruction."

Courtney Love

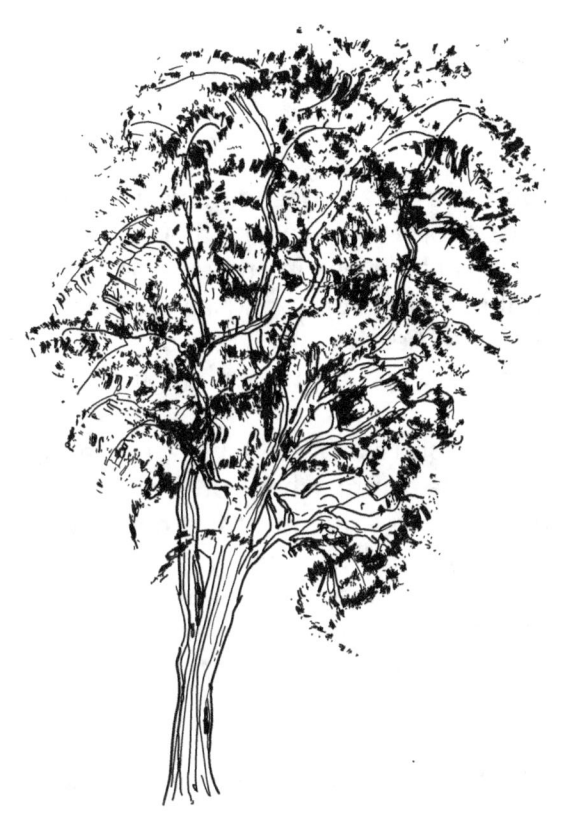

Self-Forgiveness

The act of freeing yourself from emotional bondage.

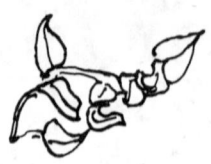

Emotions are a mode of communication your mind uses to display your reaction to an encounter, an experience, or an event. In other words, how are you feeling about what's occurring in your life at any given point in time. The trick is to be as comfortable in your unhappiness as you are in your happiness.

This might sound like double speak; however, it's an absolute truism. When you feel sad, mad, hurt, etc., take the time to identify the emotion you're experiencing as well as to arrive at an understanding of why you are having this reaction to the situation. By doing so you'll increase your emotional intelligence and the best part is that you'll come to know yourself better.

Remember that what's most important is how you see yourself.

In order to be well, allow yourself to be happy!

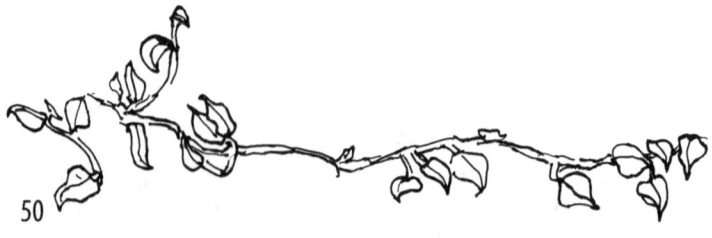

"Forgiveness ought to be like a canceled note—torn in two, and burned up, so that it never can be shown against one."

Henry Ward Beecher

"Forgive yourself for your faults and your mistakes and move on."

Les Brown

"He that cannot forgive others, breaks the bridge over which he himself must pass if he would ever reach Heaven; for everyone has need to be forgiven."

George Herbert

"There is no sense in crying over split milk. Why bewail what is done and cannot be recalled?"

Sophocles

"Forget and forgive. This is not difficult when properly understood. It means forget inconvenient duties, then forgive yourself for forgetting. By rigid practice and stern determination, it comes easy."

Mark Twain

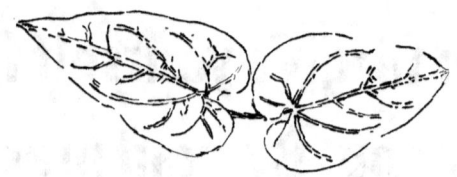

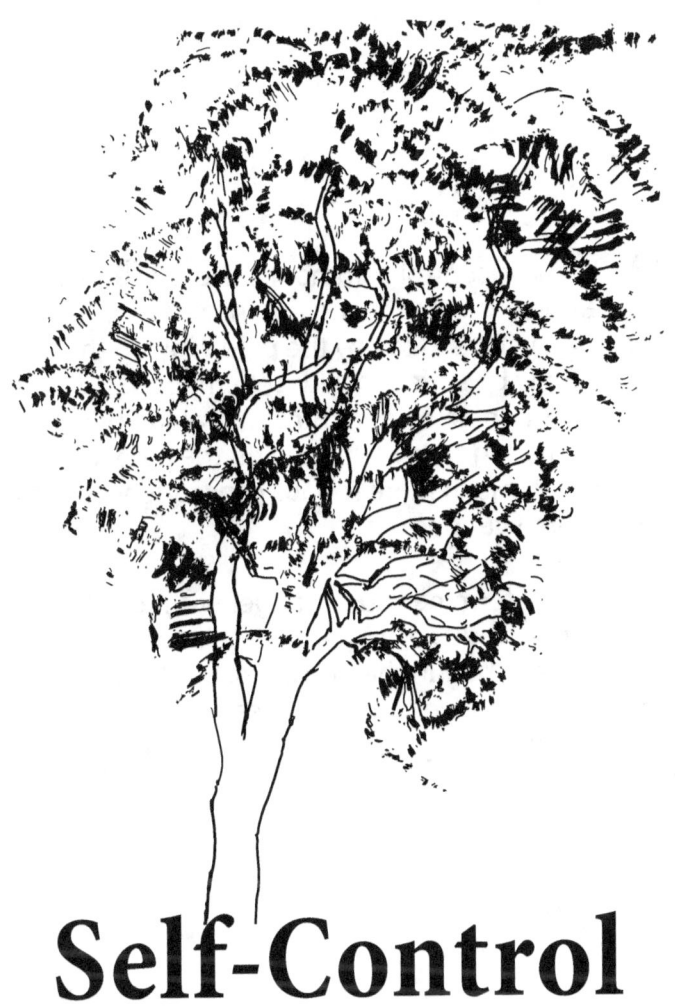

Self-Control

The acquisition of a strong aversion to negative consequences.

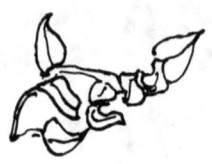

A lack of self-control commonly results in at least one unpleasant or negative consequence. In other words, you will need to pay the piper. Paying the piper might simply be suffering with self-imposed guilt for doing or not doing something or for saying or not saying something. However, paying the piper might also result in much more serious consequences such as legal ramifications.

When you determine you no longer wish to suffer the negative results of your lack of self-control, then you have begun the process of acquiring an aversion to negative consequences. This is when your behaviors will change for the better and begin to reap positive results.

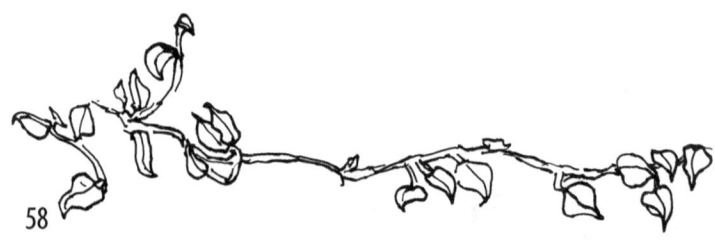

"Human nature is complex. Even if we do have inclinations toward violence, we also have inclinations to empathy, to cooperation, to self-control."

— Steven Pinker

"Self-control – what lies in our power to do, it lies in our power not to do."

Aristotle

"I cannot trust a man to control others if he cannot control himself."

Robert E. Lee

> "In that power of self-control lies the seed of eternal freedom."
>
> — *Paramahansa Yogananda*

"You are always responsible for how you act, no matter how you feel. Remember that."

Anonymous

www.ingramcontent.com/pod-product-compliance
Lightning Source LLC
Chambersburg PA
CBHW071426220526
45469CB00004B/1443